# DRY EYE
## SYNDROME RELIEF

*How to Soothe Irritated, Dry Eyes and Live Symptom-Free*

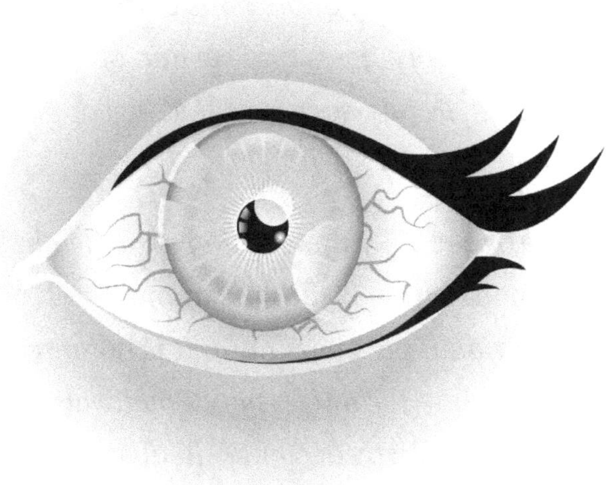

Isabella White

Title: **Dry Eye Syndrome Relief**

Author: **Isabella White**

© **2023 Isabella White. All rights reserved.**



**Disclaimer:** The information provided in this publication is for educational and informational purposes only. It is not intended as a substitute for professional medical advice, diagnosis, or treatment. Always seek the advice of your physician or qualified healthcare provider with any questions you may have regarding a medical condition.

# CONTENTS

Foreword

It is my esteemed honor to write the Foreword for Isabella White's invaluable guide to understanding and finding relief from dry eye syndrome. As an ophthalmologist who has treated thousands of patients suffering from dry, irritated eyes, I know firsthand the immense discomfort and frustration this condition can cause. The cutting-edge research and clinically proven treatments covered in this book provide much-needed answers.

Isabella's journey with chronic dry eyes sparked her passion for helping others find solutions. Her commitment to demystifying the causes and empowering readers to take control of managing this multifaceted syndrome shines through on every page. The comprehensive, practical advice in this book goes far beyond just coping; it facilitates true, lasting relief.

From explanations of tear film dynamics to targeted treatment options, Isabella equips readers with the knowledge to improve their eye health. I am confident that ***Dry Eye***

***Syndrome Relief*** will become a trusted resource for anyone seeking to understand the root factors behind their ocular irritation and inflammation. Isabella translates the latest medical findings into actionable self-care strategies anyone can benefit from.

It is my pleasure to recommend this book as essential reading for those wanting clearer, more comfortable vision. Isabella's wisdom and guidance will help you optimize your tear film, reduce environmental triggers, and make lifestyle choices that enable your eyes to feel refreshed, nourished, and protected. Find within these pages your path to living symptom-free.

**Dr. Michelle Campbell**
*Ophthalmologist and Dry Eye Specialist*
*Vision Institute of Canada*

## Preface

Blinking used to be second nature to me, just an unconscious reflex. That changed a few years ago when I started experiencing severe dryness, stinging, and burning every time my eyes opened. What began as occasional irritation progressed into a constant struggle with red, inflamed eyes that made simple tasks unbearable.

Like many, I initially tried to manage with over-the-counter drops; they provided minor relief at best. It became clear I needed to get to the root causes of why my tear film had become so dysfunctional. And I realized how little practical, patient-focused information was out there on effectively managing dry eye syndrome.

Thus began my journey to understand the science behind my symptoms. I consulted countless optometrists and ophthalmologists, reviewing all the latest research and treatments. After much trial and error, I found a multi-faceted approach that has transformed my dry eyes into healthy, lubricated eyes.

The strategies in this book combine everything I wish I knew at the start of my dry eye ordeal. I will help you understand why your eyes feel irritated and inflamed, so you can pursue targeted solutions. You'll also learn healthy habits to reduce environmental triggers and techniques to alleviate discomfort. Most importantly, you'll gain the knowledge to customize an effective management plan.

I encourage you to learn from my experience, research, and results so you can start living symptom-free. Understand the power you have to optimize your tear film, nourish your ocular surface, and breathe freely through eyelids that no longer stick and sting. This book is for anyone ready to proactively improve their eye health instead of just coping with red, dry eyes. Join me in reclaiming the freedom to open your eyes wide to the world.

**Isabella White**
*July 2023*

## Frequently Asked Questions (FAQs)

Here are answers to some frequently asked questions about dry eye syndrome.

### What causes dry eye syndrome?

Dry eyes can occur due to insufficient tear production or excessive tear evaporation. Risk factors include age, gender, medications, environmental factors, and health conditions.

### What are the symptoms of dry eye?

Common symptoms include eye irritation, redness, stinging or burning, light sensitivity, fluctuating vision, heavy eyelids, and discomfort wearing contact lenses.

### How is dry eye diagnosed?

Optometrists and ophthalmologists can diagnose dry eye through a clinical exam assessing symptoms, tear film stability, meibomian glands, and eye surface damage. They may use tests like tear osmolarity, tear breakup time, and ocular surface staining.

## How can dry eyes be treated?

Treatment aims to address the root cause and may include prescription eyedrops, tear substitutes, warm compresses, meibomian gland expression, omega-3 supplements, humidifiers, and punctal plugs. Lifestyle changes also help.

## When should someone see a doctor for dry eyes?

See an eye doctor promptly if you have severe, persistent symptoms, vision changes, eye pain or redness, corneal damage, or inadequate relief from over-the-counter treatments.

## Can dry eye syndrome cause permanent damage?

Without proper treatment, severe dry eye can result in corneal scarring, ulceration, and vision loss in extreme cases. But most symptoms can be managed with a proactive treatment regimen.

# INTRODUCTION

Dry eye syndrome is one of the most common reasons people visit eye doctors and is a frequent cause of significant irritation in our modern world. Dry eye syndrome is characterized by the feeling of grittiness, burning, stinging, and dryness in the eyes, which can be extremely uncomfortable when performing simple tasks like reading, driving, and using a computer.

This book will be your guide to understanding the causes of dry eye syndrome, the various treatment options available, and, most importantly, providing actionable advice and tips for finding relief.

You'll learn techniques to restore a healthy tear film, reduce inflammation, manage environmental factors, and soothe irritation. With the strategies in this book, you can take control of dry eye syndrome and improve the health and comfort of your eyes.

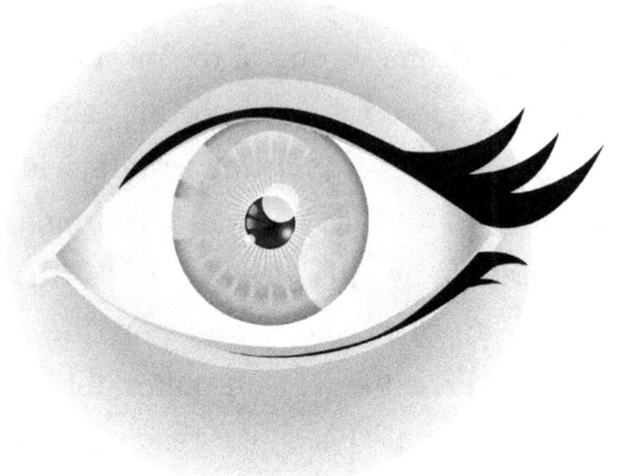

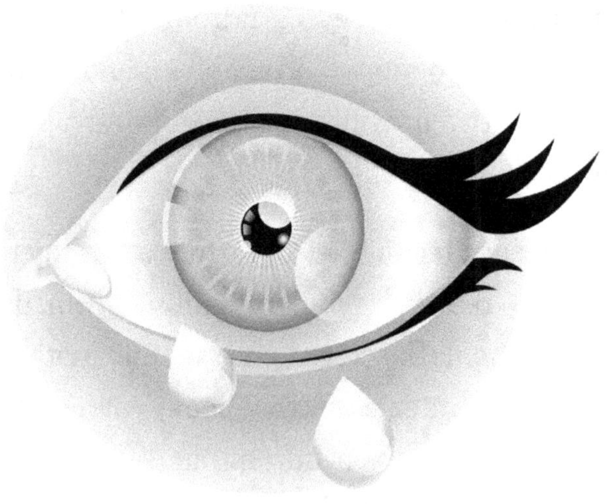

## CHAPTER ONE

# UNDERSTANDING DRY EYE SYNDROME

### What is Dry Eye Syndrome?

Dry eye syndrome is a common condition where your eyes just feel irritated and uncomfortable a lot of the time. It happens when your tears aren't able to properly lubricate and nourish your eyes. This leads to annoying sensations like dryness, stinging, grittiness, and even blurry vision.

You can think of tears as a protective layer that shields your eyes from the world. But with dry eyes, that layer gets disrupted. Your eyes end up exposed to irritation that most of us take for granted won't happen when we blink or open our eyes.

The good news is that dry eyes can be managed once you understand what's causing the problem with your tears. Let's start by looking at some of the most common symptoms.

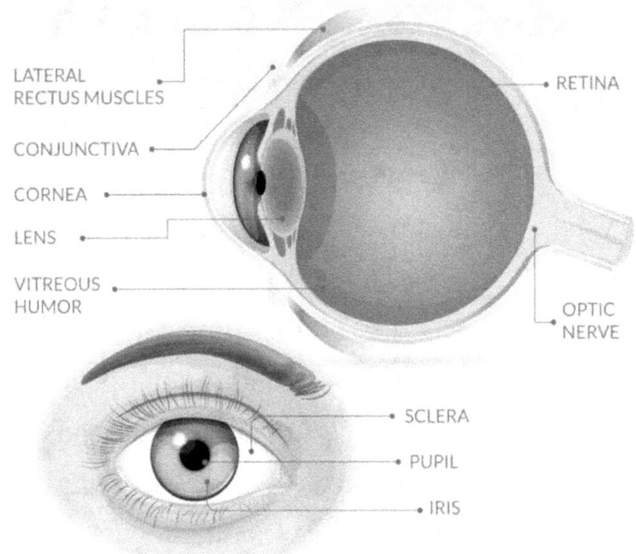


## Common Symptoms and Signs

- Dry, scratchy feeling like you have sand in your eyes
- Stinging, burning, or watery eyes
- Blurry vision that fluctuates and improves with blinking

- Redness in the whites of your eyes or on the eyelids
- Increased irritation in windy or dry environments
- Heavy eyelids, especially in the morning
- Difficulty wearing contact lenses

You may relate to some or all of these symptoms. The severity can also vary from occasional irritation to persistent discomfort. Recognizing the signs is the first step to finding relief.

## Causes and Risk Factors

There are two major causes of dysfunctional tear production:

1. **Not making enough tears:** This happens when the glands that produce the watery component don't secrete enough fluid.
2. **Losing too many tears:** This is when the oily part of your tears evaporates too quickly from the eye's surface.

Things that increase your risk of developing dry eye include:

- **Age:** Tear production can decrease as we get older.
- **Gender:** Women are more prone to dry eyes, especially after menopause.
- **Medications:** Antihistamines, birth control pills, decongestants
- **Health issues:** Autoimmune diseases, diabetes, vitamin deficiencies

## Getting Diagnosed

Seeing an optometrist or ophthalmologist is important to get an accurate dry eye diagnosis. They'll examine your eyes, ask about symptoms, and may use specialized tests to evaluate your tear film and measure tear production.

Identifying the cause of your dryness allows for more targeted treatment. The sooner you can address the root of the problem, the sooner you can find relief!

# CHAPTER TWO

# MANAGING MEIBOMIAN GLAND DYSFUNCTION

If your eyes feel dry and irritated a lot, the culprit could be dysfunction in tiny glands along your eyelids called meibomian glands. Here's what you need to know about these overlooked oil producers and how to get them working better.

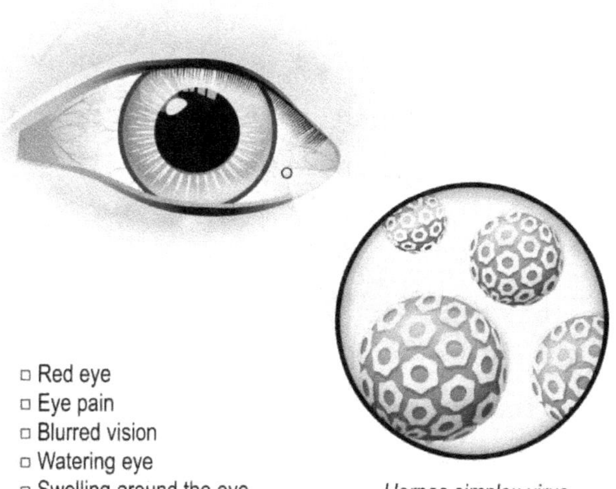

□ Red eye
□ Eye pain
□ Blurred vision
□ Watering eye
□ Swelling around the eye

*Herpes simplex virus*

## Role of Meibomian Glands in Dry Eye

Meibomian glands are specialized glands inside your upper and lower eyelids. They secrete an oily substance that forms the outer layer of your tear film. This oil prevents your tears from evaporating too quickly from the surface of your eyes.

When these glands don't function properly, you end up with an evaporative dry eye. The watery component of your tears evaporates faster than it can be replenished. This leaves your eyes parched and prone to irritation.

## Symptoms of Meibomian Gland Dysfunction

If your meibomian glands aren't secreting enough oil, symptoms may include:

- Excessive dryness and irritation, especially later in the day.
- Gritty or burning sensation in your eyes
- Blurry or fluctuating vision
- Redness and inflammation on the eyelid margins
- Crusting or debris on your lashes

Air conditioning, prolonged screen time, and other environmental factors frequently make the discomfort worse. Pay attention to these clues, as they can indicate meibomian gland problems.

## Treatment Options

There are several ways to get those sluggish meibomian glands kicked into gear:

- **Warm compresses:** Applying moist heat helps loosen the blocked oils.
- **Lid massages:** Gently massaging the eyelids can help express the oils.
- **Prescription medications:** Your eye doctor may prescribe antibiotics or anti-inflammatory drops.
- **In-office procedures:** Treatments like LipiFlow use heat and massage to unblock gland secretions.

## Meibomian Gland Expression Techniques

Manually expressing the meibomian glands can provide relief. Try gentle, repeated pressure with a warm, damp cloth on the eyelids. Or use your fingertips or a sterile cotton swab to specifically express individual glands. Just don't squeeze too hard!

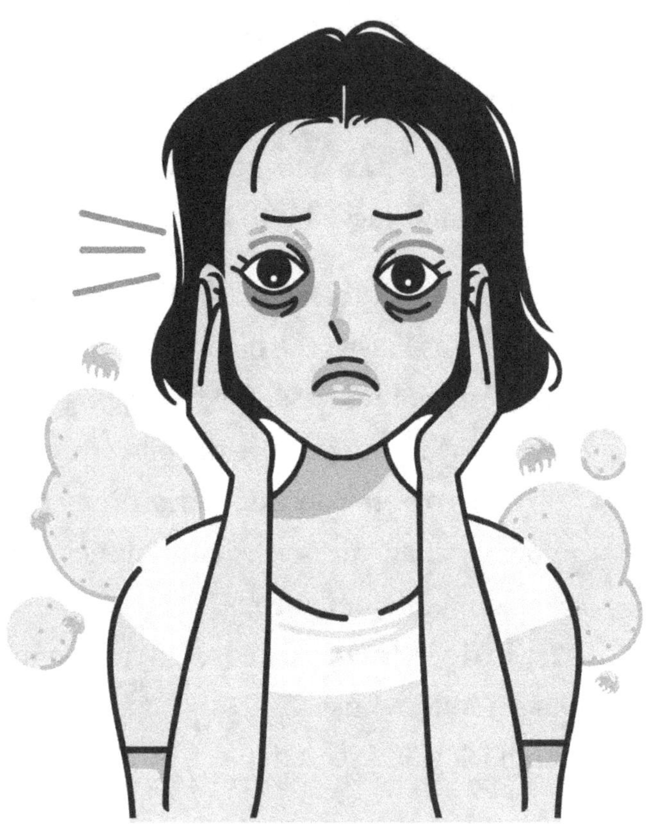

## CHAPTER THREE

# INCREASING TEAR PRODUCTION

Crying when you cut onions is one thing. But you shouldn't have to cry just trying to read emails on your computer. Let's look at how to get your eyes to make more tears.

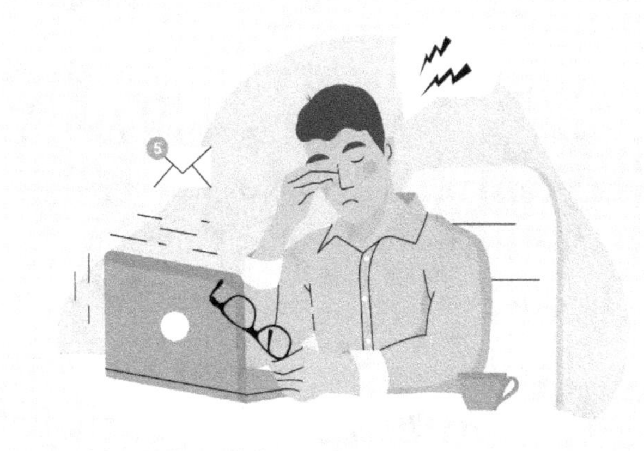

### Importance of Tear Film for Lubrication

Tears does more than just make you emotional during sappy movies. They lubricate your eyes and keep them feeling fresh. The tear film is like a protective layer of fluid that nourishes your ocular surface.

When your lacrimal glands don't secrete enough of the watery component, your eyes miss out on that lush hydration. The result is irritation, dry spots, and general discomfort.

## Pharmaceutical Treatments for Aqueous-Deficient Dry Eyes

If your dry eye is caused by inadequate tear production, prescription eye drops can help:

- **Acetylcysteine:** This mucus-thinning drop helps increase tear volume.
- **Cyclosporine:** It reduces inflammation to boost natural tear production.
- **Lifitegrast:** This newer drug dampens inflammation and stimulates tear creation.
- **Oral medications:** Pills like Xiidra or Restasis can address root causes systemically.

Work with your eye doctor to find the right prescription medication to get your tear ducts flowing freely again.

## Supplementary Tear Substitutes and Ointments

Artificial tear drops purchased over the counter lubricate the eyes and offer momentary relief. Thicker ointments coat the eyes for longer. Try different brands until you find one that soothes you.

Use drops or ointments frequently as needed; don't wait for your eyes to feel parched. Staying ahead of dryness prevents strain and damage.

## Long-term Management through Punctal Plugs

Punctal plugs are tiny devices inserted into your tear ducts to block drainage. This helps you retain more of your natural tears.

- Effective for up to 6 months before needing replacement.
- Inserted quickly and easily by an ophthalmologist
- Come in disposable, short-term, or extended-release options.

- Provide constant lubrication without eyedrop hassle!

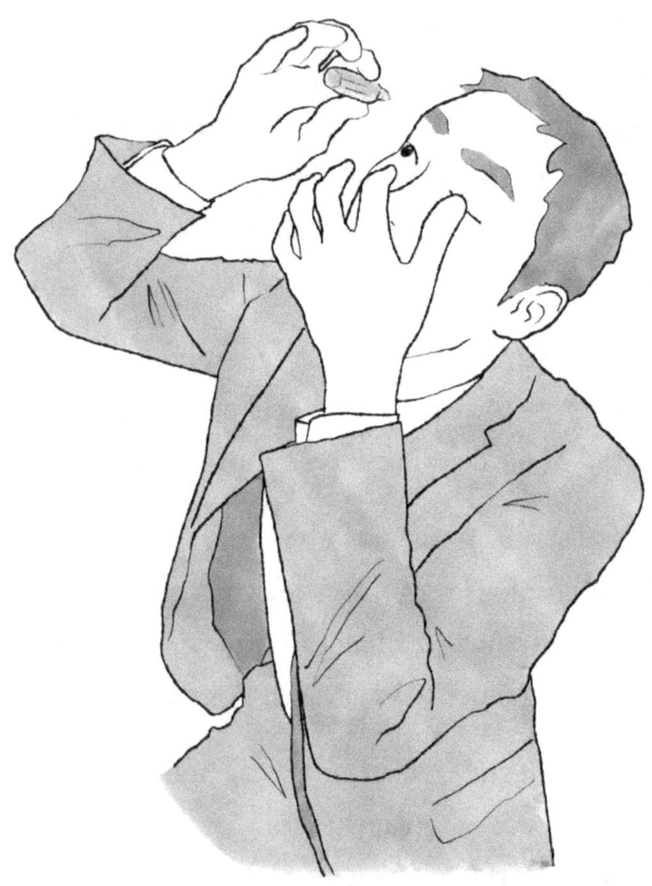

## CHAPTER FOUR

# CONTROLLING ENVIRONMENTAL FACTORS

Environmental triggers can exacerbate dry eyes. Here's how to tackle problematic indoor and outdoor conditions for happy, hydrated eyes.

### Outdoor Conditions Like Wind and Low Humidity

When heading outside, defend your eyes against:

- **Wind:** Shield your eyes with sunglasses, a hat, or by looking down.
- **Low humidity:** Carry lubricating eyedrops for quick relief in dry climates.
- **Sun:** Wear UV-blocking sunglasses to reduce sunlight exposure and drying.
- **Pollution:** Glasses create a barrier against irritants in traffic, pollen, etc.

## Indoor Factors Like Air Conditioning

To counteract drying indoor air:

- Use an air humidifier to boost moisture levels.
- Take frequent breaks from screens to blink and look off into the distance.
- Position computer monitors below eye level to minimize surface exposure when staring.
- Adjust the AC vents away from your face and stay hydrated!

## Blinking Exercises and Lid Hygiene

Keep your eyelids and the glands within them in tip-top shape:

- Clean lids daily with warm water and diluted baby shampoo.
- Apply warm compresses to loosen oil and debris.
- Practice extended blinking exercises to spread tears.
- Gently massage the lids to stimulate oil flow.

## Dietary Changes to Decrease Inflammation

Eat more omega-3 foods like fish, nuts, and avocados to reduce inflammation. And avoid inflammatory foods like gluten, dairy, alcohol, and processed carbs. Staying hydrated also helps!

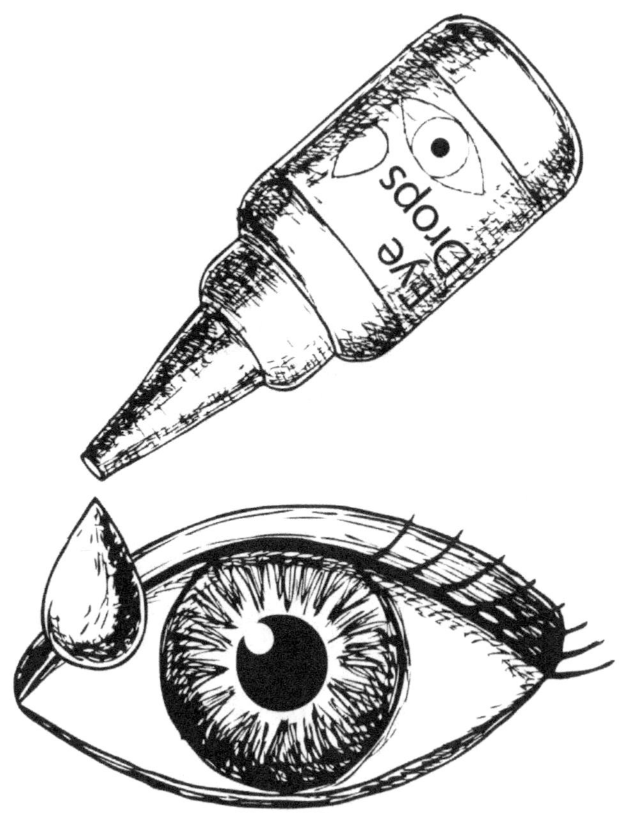

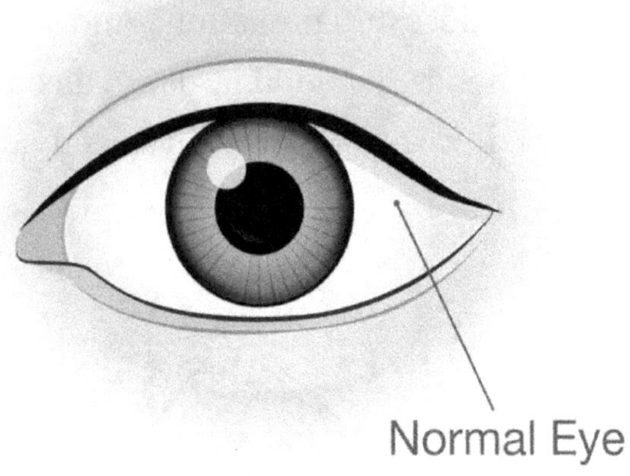

Normal Eye

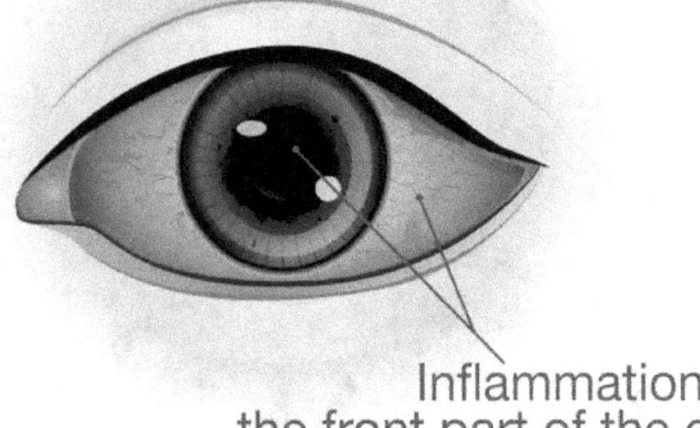

Inflammation of
the front part of the eye

## CHAPTER FIVE

# SOOTHING DRY EYE DISCOMFORT

When dry eye flares up, you need some quick symptomatic relief. Try these tips to calm the sting and redness.

### Cold Compresses, Eyewashes, and Lid Scrubs

- Chilled eye masks, cucumber slices, or damp cloths can instantly soothe.
- Eyewash rinses with soothing saline to remove irritants and hydrate the eyes.
- Foaming lid cleansers like OCuSOFT help clean crusty margins.

### Over-the-Counter Anti-Inflammatories

Redness-reducing eyedrops like Lumify contain anti-inflammatories that provide temporary relief from dry eye irritation. Just don't overuse them.

## Moisture Chamber Glasses

These specialized glasses create a humid "chamber" over your eyes, preventing tear evaporation. Wear them at night or during screen use for hydrating protection.

## Managing Digital Eye Strain

Since screens exacerbate dryness, try these tactics:

- Use artificial tear drops before and during computer use.
- Adjust font sizes for easy reading without squinting.
- Follow the 20-20-20 rule by looking away every 20 minutes for 20 seconds at 20 feet.
- Blink more! Consciously remember to blink fully while staring at screens.

## CHAPTER SIX

# WHEN TO SEE A DOCTOR

While you can manage mild dry eye yourself, severe cases may require a doctor's expertise. Here's when to seek professional help.

### Signs that Indicate a Severe Dry Eye Disease

See an ophthalmologist or optometrist promptly if you experience:

- Chronic pain, redness, and light sensitivity.
- Vision changes like blurred or fluctuating eyesight.
- **Corneal damage:** Your doctor can check for this.
- Extreme dryness with no relief from over-the-counter drops.
- Discomfort severely impacts your daily activities.

## Diagnostic Tests Like Tear Film Imaging

Your eye doctor has specialized tools to evaluate your tear film:

- **Tear breakup time:** Measures the rate of tear evaporation
- **Meibography:** Images of your meibomian glands
- **Tear osmolarity:** Assesses tear film balance
- **Corneal staining:** Checks for damage using dye drops

## Prescription Medications and Tear Duct Treatments

For moderate-to-advanced cases, doctors may prescribe:

- Stronger prescription eyedrops (steroids, biologics)
- Oral medications
- Punctal plugs retain tears by blocking ducts.
- Tear duct cauterization as a permanent drainage block

## Surgical Options for Severe Cases

If other treatments fail, options like punctal occlusion surgery may be considered to seal the tear ducts shut and prevent drainage.

Don't delay seeing an eye doctor if basic self-care isn't providing relief for your dry eyes. There are many options to give you lasting comfort!

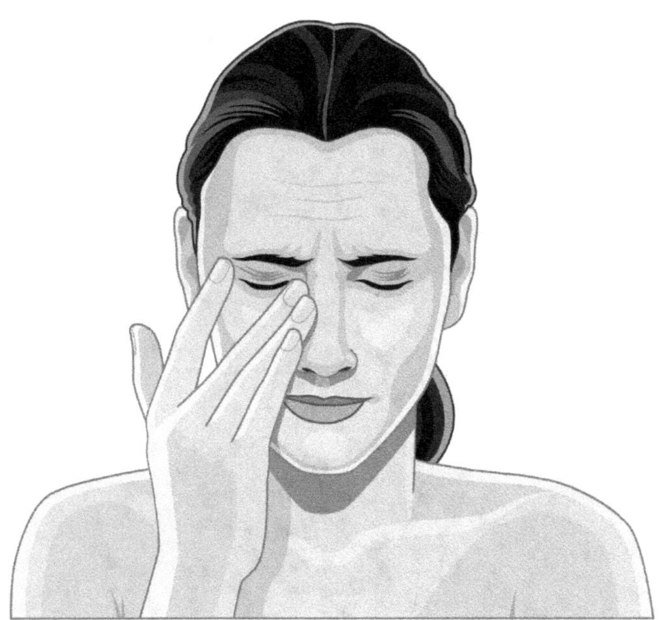

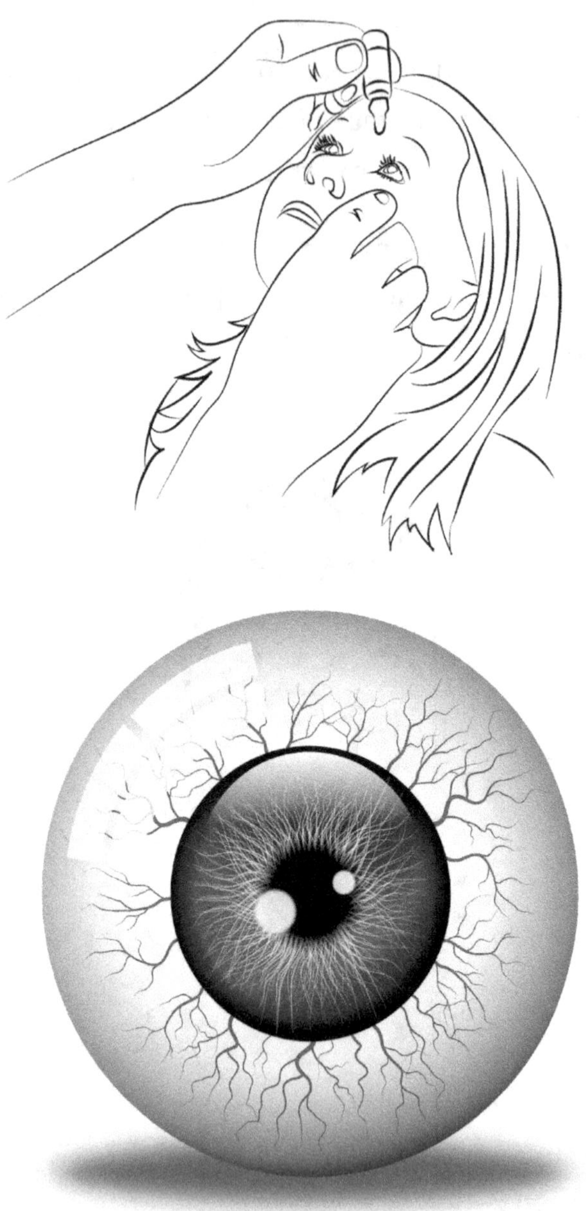

# **CONCLUSION**

Achieving Relief from Dry, Irritated Eyes

If you've picked up this book, chances are you're all too familiar with the irritating sensations of dry eye syndrome. The good news is that understanding the root causes of your dryness gives you the power to find real relief.

This book has equipped you with in-depth knowledge on managing meibomian gland dysfunction, increasing tear production, controlling environmental factors, soothing discomfort, and seeking professional care when needed.

While the treatments covered are varied, the goal is the same: reducing inflammation, optimizing your tear film, and restoring the eye comfort we all take for granted. With diligence and patience in applying the strategies suggested, you can get your eyes feeling healthy, lubricated, and irritation-free again.

I encourage you to revisit any relevant chapters as needed when flare-ups occur. Use this guide as a handy reference for maintaining happy eyes. And don't hesitate to see your eye doctor for prescribed therapies if basic self-care isn't providing sufficient relief.

You now have both the knowledge and the tools to take charge of your dry eye condition. I hope this book has provided the understanding, practical tips, and motivation you need to achieve lasting freedom from red, dry, and uncomfortable eyes. Go forth and maintain the clear, positive vision you deserve!

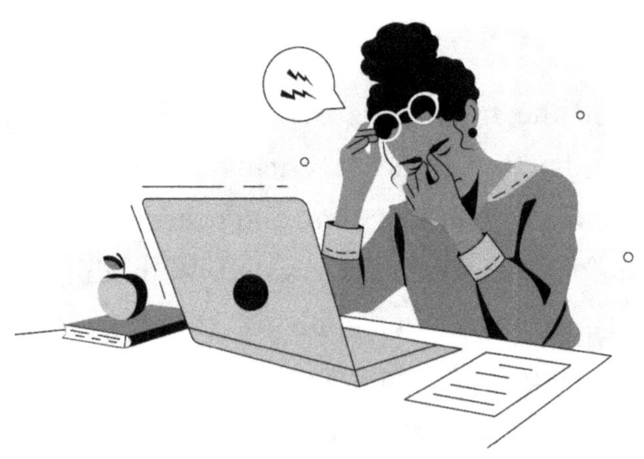

# GLOSSARY OF TERMS

**Aqueous deficiency:** Insufficient production of the watery component of tears by the lacrimal glands.

**Blepharitis:** Inflammation of the eyelids

**Cornea:** The clear, dome-shaped surface that covers the front of the eye

**Evaporative dry eye:** Excessive evaporation of tears due to meibomian gland dysfunction

**Keratoconjunctivitis sicca:** The medical name for dry eye syndrome.

**Lacrimal glands:** The glands that produce the aqueous or watery layer of tears

**Meibography:** Imaging technique to visualize the meibomian glands.

**Meibomian glands:** The oil-producing glands along the eyelid margins.

**Mucin:** The component of tears that allows them to spread evenly over the eye.

**Ophthalmologist:** Medical doctor specializing in the treatment and diagnosis of eye diseases.

**Optometrist:** Healthcare professional who examines eyes and vision disorders.

**Punctal plugs:** Tiny devices inserted into the tear ducts to block drainage.

**Tear film:** The complex, layered fluid coating the surface of the eye

**Tear osmolarity:** A measure of tear film balance

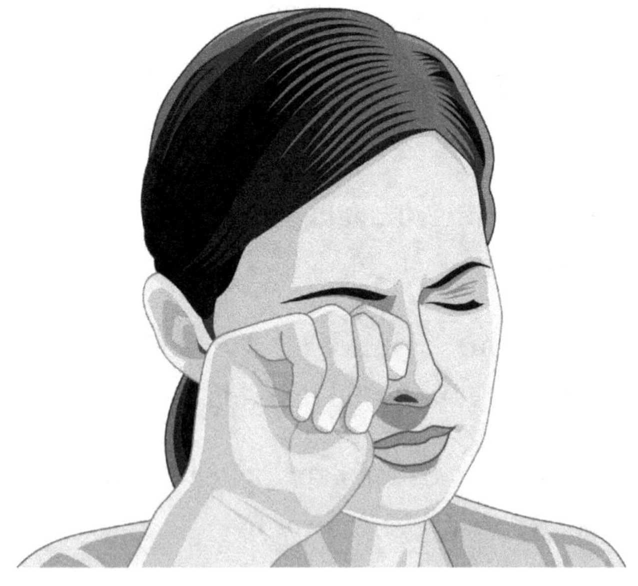

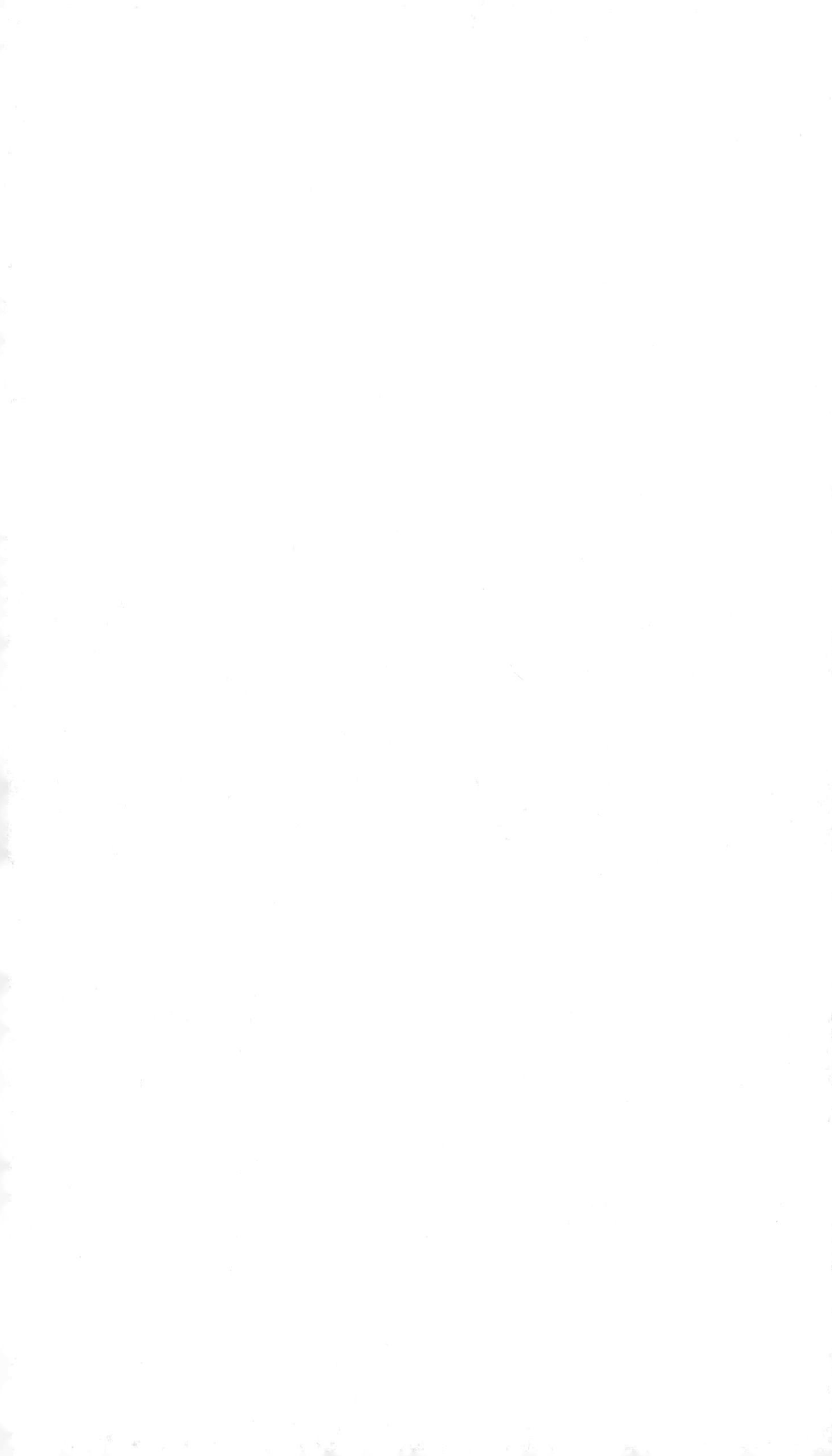